Zero Belly Cookbook

Achieve your body goals without sacrificing your enjoyment for food!

Olivia Dunham

D1445638

Introduction

Achieving your ideal weight and body takes dedication, commitment, and discipline. Aside from a well-designed and scheduled exercise routine, you will also need a well-balanced diet.

Unlike other rabbit-food diet programs, the Zero Belly diet is designed to ensure that you achieve your body goals without sacrificing your enjoyment for food. With this diet program, you'll be able to eat without restriction and even let your food watch your weight for you.

This recipe book for Zero Belly diet includes main dish, breakfast, dessert and even recipes for beverages that you can pair with your meals all throughout the day.

Oh, and did I mention desserts? Yes, desserts, but not just any ordinary dessert, chocolate desserts! For years, diet gurus have been maligning desserts as a mortal sin for dieters when it ought to be a well-deserved reward after a long day's work. Studies even show that dieters who give in to their cravings are more successful in achieving their weight goals compared to those who don't.

As a bonus, I've also listed a few teas you may want to try (if you're not already a drinker), to boost your fat melting capabilities to compliment your workout.

I hope you find this book useful in your journey to a better you.

Good luck and have fun with your Zero Belly diet!

Table of Contents

Chapter 1: Living the Zero Belly Way of Life

Losing a little over a pound a day seems like a lot to hope for, but it is achievable with the right diet, and of course, a few hours of exercise per week. The **Zero Belly diet** can help you get started by improving the health and function of your digestive system, slowing down fat tissue generation and fat storage, and building your core muscles, which prevent fatty tissue buildup and even get rid of existing excess fat.

In this chapter, we will discuss how each phase can be made possible through solid action plans and recommendations on what to eat and what to avoid.

Phase 1: Improving Your Digestive Health

The Zero Belly Diet is not just for aesthetics. Studies have shown that belly fat is linked to metabolic disorders and serious conditions like heart disease. Just as with any other diet, you start by having a healthy digestive system. Here are the steps on how to make this possible:

1. Add more (insoluble and soluble) fiber into your meals

This is one of the cornerstones of this eating regimen. Consuming healthy amounts of dietary fiber makes it easier to break down food into nutrients that blood absorbs quickly and passes along to other organs of the body.

This allows you to consume fewer calories, but with higher concentrations of essential minerals, trace elements, and vitamins. This is the true meaning of "eating less by eating more." Having healthy amounts of fiber in your diet is a valuable aid to safe, gradual, and speedy weight loss.

More importantly, when you consume fiber-rich plant-based food, your body doesn't feel hungry all the time. This lessens the possibility of you breaking your diet prematurely, craving frequently for salty/sugary/greasy food, or binging relentlessly as soon as the diet ends.

Consuming plant-based dietary fiber helps speed up toxin and waste removal by promoting easy and regular bowel movement. Having regular BM lessens: bloating, chronic flatulence, and unwanted liquid retention. This lowers risk of acquiring: compound hemorrhoids, gastric/stomach cancer, IBS or irritable bowel syndrome, and other gastrointestinal disorders. This slows down production of more adipose tissues (fat cells) too, which is great if you are trying to trim down quickly.

2. Consume little or no processed food and drinks

The Zero Belly diet advocates non-consumption of all processed food; or at the very least, severely limit intake to bare necessities.

Most processed food contains inordinately high amounts of food additives (e.g. artificial colors, flavors, enhanced nutrients, etc.), refined starches, sugar/sweeteners, salt, and preservatives.

These make food items and drinks look attractive and last longer on grocery and/or freezer shelves. This also keeps production costs down, and makes edibles highly addictive for the sake of repetitive purchases.

Health-wise, aside from being constantly linked to the development of carcinogens or cancer-producing cells in the body, chronic and prolonged consumption of processed food is the topmost reason for unwanted, and/or excessive weight gain.

Processed food and drinks contain ingredients, (namely refined starches, sugars, and sweeteners) that the gastric system mistakenly "interprets" as simple carbohydrates. These easily pass through stomach wall lining and into the bloodstream. Afterwards though, the body doesn't know how to proceed with said calories.

None of the internal organs need it. The body, which is genetically programmed to extract as much nutrients from food as possible, hoards these into adipose tissues with the intention of processing these later on. But that never happens, because calories from other food and drink keep piling up.

Unfortunately, these calories absorb a lot of electrolytes from liquids, occupy body mass, and are difficult to expend even with the most restrictive diets and physically demanding workouts.

These drain your mental and physical energy, which leads to brain fog, chronic fatigue/exhaustion, lethargy, memory loss, mental confusion, and slow metabolism. In extreme cases, these can even lower bone density, muscle tone, and immunity, increasing your risk of all forms of infections.

Additionally, poor musculature combined with weak bones can lead to early onset of lifelong degenerative bone/muscle diseases like: arthritis, sclerosis, and scoliosis.

So yes, being overweight will make you sick.

To ensure that weight loss is safely achieved in the least amount of possible time, all (or most) processed food and drinks should be off the menu for the time being. This includes:

- Alcoholic beverages
- Baked goods, pre-packed and/or commercially-manufactured confections
- Breakfast cereals
- Breakfast drinks / chocolate drinks / coffee mixes / tea mixes
- Candies and other sweets
  - Chocolate
  - Dessert mixes
  - Frozen desserts
  - Gelatin and gelatin mixes
  - Hard/soft candies
  - Marshmallows
  - Pudding
- Chips and crisps (mostly vegetable-based snack items)
- Commercially-cured meat
  - Canned meat or luncheon meat
  - Chicken nuggets
  - Deli meat
  - Ham
  - Hotdogs / sausages
- Condiments
  - Barbecue sauces
  - Catsup
  - Chili sauces / chili jellies
  - Dips
  - Margarine
  - Mayonnaise
  - Salad dressing

- Dairy-based products
  - Butter
  - Cheese
  - Cream
  - Ice cream
  - Yogurt
- Energy (granola) bars and drinks
- Fast food
- Flavored nuts, and other heavily seasoned pre-roasted nuts
- Frozen dinners and other microwavable dishes
- Instant gravy mixes, sauces and soups
- Instant noodles, and quick cooking (instant) grains
- Microwavable snacks
- Pre-mixed batter and dough
  - Brownie and cake mixes
  - Frozen cookie dough
  - Frozen pizza dough
- Processed fruits
  - Canned fruits in light/heavy syrups
  - Dried fruits and candied fruits
  - Fruit juices (ready-to-drink) and concentrates
  - Fruit sauces, jams, jellies, etc.
  - Pie fillings
- Processed vegetables
  - Canned vegetables in brine/oil/syrup
  - Pre-cut vegetables, marinated and/or seasoned
- Ready-to-cook or pre-marinated dishes
  - Hamburger mixes
- Sodas and other commercially manufactured beverages

Of course, there are exceptions to the rule. For example:

- Bacon, especially homemade bacon and other *chartercurie* are often preserved in salt and organic sweetener, like: honey and maple syrup. Avoid commercially-manufactured ones.
- Bottled capers and olives in brine or oil are acceptable.
- Canned fruits, meat and vegetables are ok as long as these are not steeped in heavy syrups and sauces. These include: canned anchovies, beans, tomatoes, tuna, etc.
- Frozen fruits and vegetables are acceptable.
- Frozen seafood is acceptable, like: fish cutlets, peeled shrimps, and pre-cut squid rings, etc.
- Homemade yogurt is ok as long as this is freshly made, and sweetened organically (no refined sugars)
- Mustard (all kinds) are highly processed, but because these contain hardly any amount of food additives and preservatives, this is still considered as safe to include in most diets, include the **Zero Belly diet**

If you have to use processed food and drinks, always opt for minimally processed ones; and use these as sparingly as possible.

3. This diet advocates non-consumption of dietary supplements

Dietary supplements should be off the menu too. These products contain overly processed ingredients that may damage your health in the long run. The risk of acquiring cancer, cardiovascular diseases, diabetes (Type II,) gastrointestinal disorders, kidney disorders, osteoporosis, and renal failure rise exponentially with long term and unsupervised use dietary supplements.

It just doesn't make sense to trade off one health concern for a far worse medical condition. It is far easier, cheaper, and healthier to just stop taking food supplements altogether.

4. Avoid sugars and sweeteners for the time being

The Zero Belly diet advocates non-consumption of sugars and sweeteners. It doesn't matter if these are organic or commercially- made, sugars and sweeteners are absorbed by the body as simple carbohydrates. High amounts of simple carbs in the bloodstream causes chronic insulin imbalance – which in turn, leads to insulin resistance or the inability of the body to process simple carbs into expendable energy.

Worse, these trigger unwanted hunger pangs, food insatiability, and cravings for greasy, salty and/or sugary food and drinks.

These physiological states are difficult to ignore, even more difficult to stop mid-way, and usually creep up on you during your unguarded moments. This is the reason why at some point, you may have consumed two liters of soda, or large bars of chocolates, or even whole cakes/pies in one sitting.

To prevent weight gain, consumption of sugars/sweeteners should be avoided or severely limited.

If you like sweets, you can always turn to fresh fruits as treats.

Green stevia, which least affects blood sugar level and has small amounts of fiber can be used to sweeten food and drinks. Do so sparingly, or only if absolutely necessary.

5. Go low-fat.

Fats and oils tend to coat stomach lining, which lessens the efficiency of gastric acids that break down food. This makes it harder for nutrients to pass through stomach walls. When this happens, the body feels deprived of vitamins and minerals. It sends out signals to your brain that it needs to consume more food – even if your stomach is already full to bursting.

Have you ever binged heavily on fatty cuts and/or deep-fried meat (e.g. cracklings, hotdogs, etc.) and still feel unsatisfied afterwards? If so, it was the large volume of grease within said items that prevented you from feeling full.

Among the different food groups, fat and oils take longest to digest. These remain in the body for relatively longer periods of time, making these the hardest to burn off and expel from the body.

To ensure weight loss, it is imperative that you consume fewer volumes of fats and oils. This will give your body more time and energy to burn off your existing ones.

If you have the means, invest in cookware that allows you to create meals without the need for additional grease. You can easily start off with buying non-stick pans, skillets or woks. Adding a steamer or steaming baskets to your kitchen tools is beneficial as well; as with non-stick grills/griller, baking dishes and sheets.

Lean meat should be on the menu (unless you are vegan or vegetarian)

The **Zero Belly diet** recommends consumption of fresh, lean meat; preferably only 3 to 6 ounces per day and only at dinner time.

Dinner should be your heaviest meal of the day. This allows your body to process proteins efficiently as you have a long "resting" period during the night; which is why you should also practice **Intermittent fasting** (more on that later.)

This also lessens that feeling of heaviness and lethargy during the day, particularly during mid-afternoon.

Eggs for breakfast are sole exceptions to this rule (more on this in the next page.)

6. Consume more water

This step seems easy, right? Not quite. Many people mistakenly believe that simply drinking more water will improve digestion. Although this statement is true, this is only half of the equation.

The other half states that you should substitute plain, unflavored water for most (if not all) of your calorific and/or processed drinks you normally take within 24 hours. This includes everything from alcoholic beverages, to coffee, to sodas, and everything else in between.

Many of these drinks are overly processed and contain high amounts of sugars and sweeteners. Some contain food additives, and preservatives which are starch-based, but hardly contain any organic or usable nutrients.

Products labeled "enriched" or "fortified" are the worst. These contain artificially-manufactured nutrients which are theoretically supposed to be good for one's health. In practice though, the body rejects these artificial enhancements, and even increases risk of triggering carcinogens.

For speedy weight loss and overall health, you should increase your daily water intake to more than 6 to 8 glasses per day (12 oz. each,) **AND** cut back on other drinks and beverages.

7. Get clean and stay clean

This is one of the hardest steps to take but it is an important element when it comes to **safe** weight loss. If possible, keep alcohol and nicotine at bay. Avoid using recreational drugs or any of the harder stuff. These can derail all your weight loss efforts.

Worse, these will seriously compromise large internal organs like: kidneys and lungs.

Phase 2: Slowing Down The Production Of Adipose Tissues

To reduce or prevent belly fat, it's important that you prevent the mechanisms that trigger the production and storage of fat, and here are some steps to achieve that.

1. Consume protein for breakfast

As counterintuitive as it sounds, it is essential to consume dense protein in the morning to slow down adipose tissue production.

Unless you are vegetarian or vegan, raw or lightly cooked eggs are highly recommended as breakfast options. Eggs are densely packed with proteins, with just the right amount of good fats to give your muscles a boost to start your day.

Eggs are also easily processed by the body, and therefore kinder to your digestive system as compared to other plant-based protein.

For the **Zero Belly diet**, you can consume up to 3 pieces of whole (but small) eggs for breakfast, or about 3 ounces. These should either be raw/partially raw (e.g. raw egg yolks, 3-minute eggs) or lightly cooked (e.g. boiled, poached, friend on dry pan, etc.)

In the interest of weight loss though, an ounce is good enough if you combine this with fresh vegetables and fruits.

If you are not partial to eggs, and have time to spare making somewhat elaborate breakfast dishes every day, you can always use fish/seafood, poultry, and red meat – though these are best suited for dinner.

Protein alternatives include 17 to 26 grams (3 ounces) of:

- ✓ Fish and seafood specifically:
    - Anchovies, canned or fresh
    - Catfish
    - Cod
    - Crab
    - Flounder
    - Grouper
    - Haddock
    - Halibut
    - Lobster
    - Mahi-mahi
    - Orange roughy
    - Perch
    - Tuna, canned or fresh
    - Salmon, canned or fresh
    - Sardines, canned or fresh
    - Scallops
    - Shrimps or prawns
    - Snapper
    - Sole
    - Swordfish
    - Tilapia
    - Trout
- ✓ Poultry, specifically:
    - Chicken
        - Breast fillets

- Leg/thigh fillets
- Cornish hen, breast fillets
- Duck, breast fillets
- Ground chicken meat, 90% lean or extra lean
- Pheasants, breast fillets
- Turkey
  - Breast fillets
  - Ground turkey meat, 90% lean or extra lean

✓ Red meat, lean cuts, specifically: beef, pork, and veal
- Beef and veal
  - Arm roast
  - Bottom round
  - Bottom round steak
  - Chuck shoulder roast
  - Cured meat
    - Beef jerky
    - Corned beef
    - Pastrami
  - Flank steak
  - Ground beef, 95% lean or extra lean
  - Ground veal, 90% lean or extra lean
  - Leg cuts
  - Pepperoni
  - Rib eye
  - Round eye
  - Round tip
  - Rump roast
  - Sirloin tip

- Tenderloin
- Tenderloin steak
- Top loin
- Top sirloin
- Top round steak
- Veal arm steak
- Veal blade
- Veal cutlet

- Lamb
  - Arm
  - Arm chop
  - Boneless chops
  - Fore shanks
  - Ground lamb, 90% lean or extra lean
  - Leg
  - Leg roast
  - Loin
  - Loin chops
  - Shanks
  - Tenderloin
- Pork
  - Center loin
  - Center loin chops
  - Cured meat
    - Canadian bacon
    - Ham
    - Pepperoni
    - Pork jerky
  - Ground pork, 95% lean or extra lean
  - Loin rib chop

- Rib chop, bone-in and boneless
- Sirloin roast, bone-in and boneless
- Tenderloin
- Top loin
- Top loin chops
- Top loin roast
- Pork butt/shoulder, trimmed well
- Pork chop

- Wild game, e.g. bison, elk, rabbit, reindeer, and venison
  - Shanks
  - Tenderloin

Low fat cow's milk, goat's milk, and sheep's milk, which contain 2% fat and sugar-free, are viable sources of dense protein in the morning. Serve these plain, about 8 grams or less than 1 cup per serving. Or, incorporate milk in reduced portions with fresh fruit/vegetable shakes or smoothies.

Vegan and vegetarian options include:

- ✓ Beans, 14 to 17 grams (¾ to 1 cup, loosely packed) of:
  - Black beans
  - Broad *(fava)* beans
  - Garbanzos or chick peas
  - Lima beans
  - Mung beans
  - Navy beans
  - Kidney beans
  - White beans

- ✓ Green peas, 4 to 9 grams, (¾ to 1 cup, loosely packed)
- ✓ Non-dairy milk substitutes, 6 to 9 grams (1 cup) of:
    - Almond milk
    - Cashew milk
    - Coconut milk
    - Flax milk
    - Hazelnut milk
    - Hemp milk
    - Macadamia milk
    - Oat milk
    - Quinoa milk
    - Rice milk
    - Walnut milk
- ✓ Raw nuts and seeds, 4 to 9 grams (1 ounce) of:
    - Almonds
    - Chia seeds
    - Flax seeds
    - Lentils
    - Peanuts
    - Pistachios
    - Pumpkin seeds
    - Quinoa
    - Squash seeds
    - Sunflower seeds
    - Watermelon seeds

2. Consume more fresh produce

The **Zero Belly diet** advocates consumption of more fresh produce, particularly, organic fruits and vegetables. Aside from their high-fiber content, these usually contain only small amounts of fats, almost no salt and relatively low amounts of sugar.

You can consume relatively larger volumes (in moderation, of course) without packing on the pounds. Consuming raw fruits and vegetables is highly recommended; but lightly cooked ones are also acceptable.

Avoid eating vegetable-based dishes that are heavily steeped in gravies and sauces, or those that are deep-fried, or swimming in butter or grease.

3. No to soy

For the time being, avoid consuming soy and all soy-based products.

Although soy is being touted as a healthier alternative to most meats, these are also heavily processed, artificially flavored, and choked to the gills with preservatives. The body has a harder time processing these, and can contribute to the production of more adipose tissues.

Even if you are vegetarian or vegan, it is best to avoid soy-based products while following the **Zero Belly diet**.

Avoid: *miso, natto,* soybean, soybean flour, soymilk, soy nuts, soybean paste (fermented ones too,) soybean oil, soy ice cream, soy sauce, soy yogurt, sweet bean sauce, *tempeh*, teriyaki sauce, textured vegetable protein, tofu and tofu skins.

Fresh *edamame* cooked in its pod is okay, as this is often considered as vegetable.

4. Eat in moderation

This diet is all about consuming more nutrients. It is not, however, a license to binge and overindulge at every meal. Although the **Zero Belly diet** is not quite restrictive, *it is still not advisable to eat large volumes of food, and drink copiously all the time, every time.*

It is best to consume 3 small meals per day, and 2 even smaller snacks in between. Make sure that you consume less than 2,000 calories per day just to ensure that you lose weight as fast as possible.

Add more raw leafy greens (and some edible flowers, fruits, herbs and spices) to your meals. If fact, without the addition of heavy dressings and vinaigrettes, you can consume all the salad greens that you can hold. Simple dips like citrus juice or vinegar with pinch of salt and black pepper is acceptable though.

The best ones to consume are:

- Arugula or rocket
- Baby beet greens
- Baby spinach leaves
- *Bak choi*
- Basil leaves
- Belgian chicory or French endive
- Bell peppers
- Bibb, Boston or butter head lettuce
- Blood orange

- Butter crunch lettuce
- Cabbage: green, red (purple,) and white
- *Calamond in / calamansi*
- Celery
- Chervil
- Chili peppers
- Chives
- Cilantro/coriander
- Clementine
- Cucumber
- Cress: curly cress, land, upland cress, and watercress
- Dill
- Dandelion greens, young tender stems
- Escarole or broad leafed endive
- Fennel
- Fenugreek
- Field salad or lamb's lettuce
- Frisée or curly endive
- Garlic chives
- Grapefruit
- Iceberg lettuce
- Japanese greens or *mizuna*
- *Jicama*
- Kaffir lime
- Key lime
- Kumquat
- *Kinnow*
- Leeks
- Lemon
- Lemon thyme
- Lime
- Loose leaf lettuce: red and green

- Marjoram
- Mandarin orange
- Mint
- Napa cabbage
- Oak leaf lettuce: red and green
- Orange
- Oregano
- Parsley
- Peppermint
- Persian lime
- Pomelo
- Radicchio
- Romaine lettuce or cos
- Rosemary
- Satsuma
- *Shiso*
- Swiss chard
- Tangelo
- Tangerine
- Tatsoi
- Thai basil
- Thyme
- Tomatoes

Other than water, and the occasional liquid meal replacements (recipes included in last chapter,) it is recommended that you limit your sugar-free beverage intake to only 2 cups (4 to 6 oz. only) per day. Acceptable options are limited to: (dried, loose leaf and powdered green) tea, and brewed coffee (not instant). These should all be dairy and sugar-free.

5. Yes to fat-burning food

Include more organic ingredients to your meals that process stored calories into expendable energy. These include:

- Almonds and almond butter
- Apple
- Apple cider vinegar
- Asparagus
- Avocado
- Beans
- Berries
- Broccoli
- Brown rice
- Butternut squash
- Cantaloupe
- Carrots
- Cayenne pepper
- Chili / hot pepper
- Cinnamon
- Citruses, particularly lemons, limes and oranges
- Coconut and coconut by-products, like butter and oil
- Coffee, brewed, use sparingly
- Cottage cheese, rinsed, drained
- Dark chocolate
- Eggs
- Extra virgin olive oil
- Flaxseed
- Garlic
- Ginger
- Greek yogurt
- Green leafy vegetables

- Green tea leaves and *matcha* powder
- Lean red meat
- Legumes
- Lentils
- Mushrooms
- Mustard
- Oolong tea
- Pear
- Peas
- Pine nuts
- Quinoa
- Salad greens (see list from previous page)
- Salmon
- Spices
- Spinach
- Steel-cut oats
- Stinging nettle
- Sweet potato
- Taro
- Tomatoes
- Tuna
- Unsalted nuts
- Walnuts
- Watermelon
- Whole grains
- Yam

Phase 3: Strengthening Core Muscles To Help Burn Off Existing Or Excess Belly Fats

Muscles enhance metabolism as they need more calories to maintain. That's why you're going to need to boost your core muscles. Here's how.

1. Fast for 8 to 12 hours each day

To help speed things along, the **Zero Belly diet** recommends intermittent fasting. Other than digestion, this allows the body to focus on other autonomic bodily functions such as bone regeneration, cell renewal, and healing. This is also the time when core muscles are developed and strengthened.

Daily fasting period should begin 2 hours after dinner or after your last food/beverage intake. It should end 8 to 12 hours later. As a novice in the **Zero Belly diet**, you can start off with 6 hours of fasting per night for the first week.

Gradually increase your fasting period to 8 hours or longer. However, it is imperative that you extend your fasting period gradually. If your body feels starved in the morning, your tendency is to either gorge on greasy or sugary food/drinks as soon as you wake up, or overeat the night before. Both of which will prevent you from losing weight quickly.

To avoid this:

- ✓ **Start small.** 6 hours of fasting during the night shouldn't pose any physical hardship to anyone. This is usually the time you dedicate to sleep anyway. But this means that you have to avoid midnight fridge raids, and those nibbles between dinner and bedtime.

✓ **Set and follow a specific schedule.** Your fasting should begin and end at a specific time. This gives your body a routine to follow, which makes it easier on your digestion.

✓ **No calories.** Drinking plain water or munching on shave ice/ice cubes is acceptable within said time frame, as these have absolutely no calories.

✓ **Get enough restive sleep.** Getting quality sleep is one of the best ways of losing unwanted pounds, without (literally!) lifting a finger. 6 to 8 hours of snoozing can burn off as much energy as taking a brisk walk through the neighborhood for 5 minutes.

This prolonged resting period works wonder for all the involuntary functions of the body including: digestion, transmittal of nutrients to different parts of the body, waste removal, bone knitting, and development of muscles.

Something to remember: studies show that when you eat fewer calories at dinner, you get longer and more restive sleep at night.

2. Subscribe to an active lifestyle

Before you think about body sculpting, and creating those abdominal 6-packs, you need to trim down and really lose some weight. You cannot do that if you spend all day sitting on the couch, or parked in front of the computer.

At this point, any exercise will do: brisk walking for 15 minutes, cycling to and from work, swimming for an hour a day, and even taking up dancing lessons once a week. Any physical activity will help you trim down in a hurry.

To increase your weight loss endeavors though, it is essential that you burn off just as much (or more) calories than what you consume. Low impact exercises are easy to do and can really burn off stored calories in a hurry.

These include:
- Boxing classes
- Cross-country skiing
- Cycling
- Dancing
- Golf
- Hiking
- Kayaking
- Kettle bell exercises
- Pilates
- Rock climbing
- Rollerblading
- Snow shoeing
- Step aerobics
- Strength-training (beginner's level)
- Swimming
- *Tai chi*
- Total body resistance exercises
- Trampoline jumping / rebounding
- Walking and brisk walking
- Water aerobics
- Working on the elliptical machine
- Working on the rowing machine

- Working on the stair master
- Yoga
- Zumba

Chapter 2: Breakfast

Eggs Benedict

Enjoy a guilt-free savory breakfast that is packed with protein to keep you filled and energized to start your day.

Ingredients:

- 2 English muffins (gluten-free), split in half

- 2 cups of packed spinach leaves

- 4 eggs

- 2 tablespoons of mayonnaise

- Olive oil cooking spray

- Smoked paprika

Cooking Directions:

1. Toast the English muffins until it becomes golden brown.

2. Poach the eggs.

3. Prepare a medium pan and set over medium heat. Spray with the olive oil cooking spray and add in the spinach leaves. Cook the spinach and use a rubber spatula to stir the spinach. Once wilted, transfer the

spinach on a plate covered with paper towels to remove any excess water.

4. Divide the spinach into 4 equal portions and place each on top of the toasted muffins. Then, place one egg and ½ tablespoon of mayonnaise on top of the each muffin. Sprinkle a bit of smoked paprika for added taste.

This recipe is good for 4 servings.

Blueberry Good Breakfast

A staple breakfast reinvented into a high-fiber and high-protein meal.

Ingredients:

For the syrup

- ¼ cup of fresh blueberries

- 2 tablespoons of water

- 2 tablespoons of maple syrup

For the pancakes

- 2 cups of oat flour

- ¼ teaspoon of kosher salt

- 1 tablespoon of baking powder

- 1 cup of unsweetened almond milk

- 1 egg

- ½ tablespoon of extra-virgin olive oil

- ½ teaspoon of vanilla extract

- 2 egg whites, whipped until soft peaks form

- Juice of ½ lemon

- Olive oil cooking spray

- ½ cup of fresh blueberries

Cooking Directions:

1. Prepare a small saucepan and set over medium heat. Add the water, maple syrup and blueberries into the pan to make the blueberry syrup. Bring the mixture to a low simmer and cook for 5 minutes while stirring occasionally. Set aside.

2. Prepare a griddle and set over medium heat.

3. In a mixing bowl, combine the baking powder, salt and oat flour.

4. In another mixing bowl, whisk together the olive oil, almond milk, vanilla extract, egg and lemon juice.

5. Gradually add in the flour mixture into the second mixing bowl and mix until the ingredients are just combined. Fold in the egg whites gently into the mixture.

6. Spray the griddle with olive oil cooking spray and use a ¼ cup measure to add the pancake batter on the pan. Cook for 2 minutes and place a couple of blueberries on top before flipping to cook the other side. Cook for another 2 minutes. Do the same procedure until all of the pancake batter is used up.

7. Divide the pancakes into 4 servings and place it on serving plates. Top with the blueberry syrup and a couple of blueberries if you have extra.

This recipe is good for 4 servings.

Fresh Mexican Omelet

A breakfast you will want to jump out of bed for.

Ingredients:

- 1 cup of canned pinto beans, drained then rinsed

- 3 whole eggs

- Juice of ½ lime

- 5 egg whites

- ½ cup of guacamole

- ½ cup of salsa

- Olive oil cooking spray

Cooking Directions:

1. Add the lime juice and pinto beans to a food processor. Pulse until the mixture resembles refried beans.

2. Prepare a small, non-stick pan and coat with olive oil cooking spray. Set over medium heat.

3. Whisk together the egg whites and whole eggs. Divide the egg mixture into 4 equal portions. Pour the first part on the pan. Using a spatula, draw the egg to the center of the pan to let the uncooked egg slide under.

4. Once the egg has set, take a quarter of the bean mixture and spoon down the center of the omelet. Use a spatula

to fold over a third of the omelet to cover the mixture. Take the omelet from the pan and transfer on a plate, flipping on the last second to form a folded omelet.

5. Place a tablespoon of guacamole on top and 2 tablespoons of salsa.

6. Repeat the same procedure with the remaining ingredients.

This recipe is good for 4 servings.

Mushroom and Eggs

Getting tired of having the same thing every morning? This recipe will give a tasty twist on your first meal of the day.

Ingredients:

- 1 large cap of Portobello mushroom

- Salt

- Pepper

- ½ tablespoon of olive oil, divided

- 1 egg

- ⅛ avocado, sliced thinly

- 2 egg whites

Cooking Directions:

1. Preheat broiler. Prepare a large baking sheet and line with tin foil.

2. Remove the stem from the mushroom and discard. Use half of the olive oil to brush the mushroom cap on both sides. Then, place the mushroom cap on the baking sheet with the gill-side facing up.

3. Place the baking sheet in the broiler and broil the mushroom for 5 minutes. Turn the mushroom to cook the other side and return to the broiler and broil for another 5 minutes.

4. Prepare a medium pan and set over medium-low heat. Add in the remaining olive oil.

5. Whisk the egg and egg whites together and pour it into the pan to make scrambled eggs. When the eggs are just set, remove the pan from the heat. Place the scrambled eggs in the mushroom cap and add the avocado slices on top. Use salt and pepper to season accordingly.

This recipe is good for 1 serving.

Hot Breakfast

Looking for something spicy to wake you up this morning? This hot breakfast will surely chase your sleepiness away.

Ingredients:

- 1 can of black beans, drained then rinsed

- Hot sauce

- Juice of 1 lime

- 4 eggs

- Salt and pepper

- 4 egg whites

- 4 tablespoons of prepared salsa

- ½ avocado, sliced

Cooking Directions:

1. Add the lime juice, black beans and a dash of hot sauce in a food processor and pulse. Prepare a small pan and set over medium heat. Lightly coat with cooking spray.

2. Beat one egg and one egg white together in a mixing bowl. Season with pepper and salt and whisk together. Add the mixture into the pan. Using a spatula, stir and lift the cooked egg to let the raw eggs slide underneath.

3. When the eggs are just set, place a quarter of the black bean mixture on the center of the omelet. Fold about a third of the omelet over the mixture and take the omelet from the pan. Slide the omelet on a plate, flipping on the last second, to make one rolled omelet. Place ¼ of the salsa and a couple of avocado slices on top.

4. Repeat the same procedure with the remaining ingredients.

This recipe is good for 4 servings.

Berry Breakfast Bowl

Here is a new way to add your favorite peanut butter to your everyday meal.

Ingredients:

- 1 cup of water

- 1 tablespoon of natural peanut butter

- ½ cup of quick-cooking oats

- ½ cup of strawberries

Cooking Directions:

1. Fill a small saucepan with water and bring to a boil.

2. Once the water is boiling, add in the oats and stir. Cook for 3 minutes.

3. Before removing the saucepan from heat, add in the strawberries and peanut butter into the oats and stir.

4. Serve while still warm.

This recipe is good for 1 serving.

Stir-Fried Quinoa with Quail Eggs

This grain-free fried rice is loaded with vegetables. If you are not a fan of quail eggs, substitute 2 small hardboiled eggs instead. Peel these and roughly chop.

Ingredients:

- 1 tablespoons extra virgin olive oil

- 1 cup cooked quinoa, cooked according to package instructions

- 1 tablespoon minced garlic

- 1 piece shallot, peeled and minced

- 8 pieces, hardboiled quail eggs, peeled and halved lengthwise

- 1 cup mixed frozen vegetables (carrots, corn and peas,) thawed

- Salt and black pepper

- 2 cups, packed, napa cabbage, julienned

- 1 cup, packed red cabbage, cored, julienned

- 1 generous pinch chives, minced

Cooking Directions:

1. Pour oil into wok set over medium heat.

2. Sauté onion and garlic until former turns transparent.

3. Except for quail eggs and parsley, add remaining ingredients into wok. Stir-fry until well combined. Taste. Season with salt and pepper.

4. Continue cooking for 5 to 7 minutes or until cabbage becomes limp.

5. Turn off heat. Serve dish in large platter. Garnish with fresh parsley and quail egg halves. Serve warm.

This recipe is good for 4 to 6 servings.

Chapter 3: Lunch Options

Perfect Lunch Soup

Not feeling well? This soup will get you up and running in no time.

Ingredients:

- 1 tablespoon of olive oil

- 2 cloves of garlic, minced

- 1 medium onion, minced

- 1 tablespoon of fresh ginger, skin removed and minced

- 2 medium carrots, skin removed and diced

- ½ jalapeno, minced

- 1 cup of dried green lentils

- 1 bay leaf

- ¼ teaspoon of cumin

- 1 can of light coconut milk

- 1 tablespoon of soy sauce (reduced sodium)

- 3 cups of vegetable stock (low sodium)

- Salt and pepper

- Chopped cilantro

Cooking Directions:

1. Prepare a medium pot and set over medium heat. Add in the olive oil.

2. Once the oil is hot, add in the ginger, onion, garlic, carrots and jalapeno. Sauté for 3 minutes or until the onions become translucent and soft.
3. Add the cumin, lentils, coconut milk, bay leaf and vegetable stock into the pot. Reduce the heat to low and simmer for 30 minutes or until the lentils become tender.

4. Add the soy sauce and season the soup using the pepper and salt. If you want, you can also puree the soup using a blender for thicker consistency. Garnish with chopped cilantro before serving.

This recipe is good for 6 servings.

Mayo-Free Waldorf Salad

Fruit, nutty, and healthy – what more could you possibly ask from a quick-fix, but filling fresh salad?

Ingredients:

- 2 small red apples, cored and diced

- 2 small green apples, cored and diced

- 4 celery stalks, diced

- ¼ cup dark raisins

- ¼ cup golden raisins

- ¼ cup, loosely packed, roasted walnuts, chopped

- 3 tablespoons walnut oil

- 1 tablespoon apple cider vinegar

- 1 tablespoon fresh lime juice

- Pinch of salt and pepper

Preparation:

1. Whisk apple cider vinegar, lime juice, pepper, salt and walnut oil in a bowl until salt dissolves. Taste. Adjust dressing's seasoning if needed.

2. Place remaining ingredients in salad bowl, including dressing. Toss to combine.

3. Serve at room temperature or slightly chilled.

This recipe is good for 4 servings.

Pear and Almonds on Bed of Greens

Basically, all you need to do for this quick lunch option is to toast some nuts, cut up a fruit, prep some salad greens, and pour in a few tablespoons of dressing.

Ingredients:

- 1 large pear, cored, halved lengthwise, thinly sliced into half-moons

- ¼ cup blanched almond slivers, toasted on dry pan, cooled

- 1 large head iceberg lettuce, cored, leaves separated

- 1 cup loosely packed dandelion greens

- 1 cup loosely packed baby spinach leaves

- 3 sprigs parsley leaves and tender stems

- 3 tablespoons extra virgin olive oil

- 2 tablespoon lemon juice, freshly squeezed

- Pinch of salt and pepper

Preparation:

1. Whisk lemon juice, oil, pepper, and salt in a bowl until dressing comes together.

2. Rinse and spin-dry iceberg lettuce leaves, dandelion greens, spinach leaves and parsley. Roughly tear these apart into bite-sized pieces. Place these into a salad bowl along with sliced pears and dressing. Toss to combine.

3. Sprinkle almonds on top. Serve immediately.

This recipe is good for 4 to 6 servings.

Guilt-Free Tuna Salad

Tuna salad has always been a staple in lunch menus, but this spicy recipe helps burn off unwanted fats as well.

Ingredients:

- 1 (6 oz.) can tuna chunk in oil, drain lightly

- 2 tablespoons lemon juice, freshly squeezed

- 2 tablespoons Dijon mustard

- 2 heaping tablespoons raisins

- 1 6-inch celery stalk, minced

- 1 large cucumber, ends and seeds removed, diced

- 1 large onion, minced

- 1 banana chili, deseeded, minced

- Pinch of salt, pepper and Spanish paprika

- 8 to 12 whole endive leaves (Belgian chicory,) bottoms trimmed, add as many as you want

Preparation:

1. Except for endive leaves, combine remaining ingredients in a bowl. Mix until well incorporated. Taste. Add more salt and pepper if desired.

2. Place equal portions of salad into single-serve bowls, with 2 (or more) endive leaves. Serve. Use endives as edible spoons.

This recipe is good for 4 to 6 servings.

Melon Salad with Cashew Nuts

Tuna salad has always been a staple in lunch menus, but this spicy recipe helps burn off unwanted fats as well.

Ingredients:

- 2 sprigs fresh mint, roughly torn

- 1½ pounds red watermelon, visible seeds removed, cubed

- 1½ pounds yellow watermelon, visible seeds removed, cubed

- 1 medium grapefruit, pulp only, pips removed, cubed

- ¾ cup store-bought roasted cashew nuts, lightly salted

- Salt, optional

Preparation:

1. Place grapefruits, red watermelon and yellow watermelon in large salad bowl. Gently toss to combine. Chill for at least 1 hour before serving.

2. Sprinkle in remaining ingredients. Toss gently.

3. Taste. Add more salt if desired. Serve.

This recipe is good for 4 to 6 servings.

Avocado and Quinoa Salad

Avocado is quite versatile. This can be incorporated in dishes, drinks, and dips. In salads, avocadoes provide creaminess with the right amount of fat.

Ingredients:

- 2 cups cooked red quinoa, forked through

- 1 tablespoon balsamic vinegar

- 1 small lime, zested and juiced, pips removed

- 1 large cucumber, ends trimmed, halved, deseeded, diced

- 1 large shallot, julienned

- 1 large just ripe avocado, peeled, pitted, diced

- ½ cup loosely packed dill fronds, roughly chopped

- ½ cup loosely packed blanched almond flakes, toasted on dry pan, cooled

- ½ cup loosely packed fresh cilantro, minced

- ¼ pound red radishes, tops and bottoms trimmed, sliced paper-thin

- Extra virgin olive oil for drizzling

- Salt and white pepper

Preparation:

1. Place ingredients in large salad bowl. Gently toss to combine.

2. Taste. Add more olive oil, or salt or white pepper if desired.

3. Serve.

This recipe is good for 4 to 6 servings.

Lentils in Vegetable Soup

This recipe is filling, rich in nutrients, and economical to make. Make large batches of this soup, freeze leftovers, and reheat as needed over the stovetop or in microwave oven.

Ingredients:

- 1 tablespoon coconut oil

- 1 large bunch of fresh kale, stems removed, sliced into ½-inch thick strips

- 1 generous pinch fresh thyme, roughly chopped

- 2 cups brown or red lentils

- 4 large leeks, roots trimmed, minced

- 6 cups vegetable or mushroom stock, unsalted

- 15 ounce canned button mushrooms, pieces and stems, drained lightly

- 28 ounce canned whole tomatoes, drained lightly

- Salt and white pepper

Preparation:

1. Pour oil into Dutch oven set over medium heat.

2. Sauté leeks until soft, about 3 minutes.

3. Pour in canned tomatoes. Stir often, breaking up and/or crushing tomatoes as you go.

4. Pour in remaining ingredients. Bring soup to a boil. Secure lid. Simmer soup for 30 minutes or until lentils are fork-tender.

5. Turn off heat. Taste. Add more salt and pepper if desired. Serve warm.

This recipe is good for 6 servings.

Broccoli Soup

This toothsome soup is so easy to make. Whip this up on hectic days.

Ingredients:

- ½ cup raw cashew nuts

- 1 large sweet potato, peeled, diced

- 1 large sweet onion, minced

- 2 pounds fresh broccoli, include florets, leaves and stems, tough parts removed, roughly chopped

- 4 cups vegetable or mushroom broth, low-sodium

- 4 large garlic cloves, peeled, grated

- Cayenne powder

- Salt and white pepper

Preparation:

1. Pour ingredients into Dutch oven set over high heat. Stir. Bring to boil. Secure lid. Simmer soup for 30 minutes or until lentils are fork-tender.

2. Turn off heat. Using an immersion blender, process soup until smooth.

3. Taste. Add more cayenne powder, salt and pepper if desired. Serve warm.

This recipe is good for 4 servings.

Steak and Frites
Classic steakhouse recipe that is both sumptuous and healthy.

Ingredients:

For the frites

- 1 lb of Russet potatoes

- ½ teaspoon of dried thyme

- 1 tablespoon of extra-virgin olive oil

- ½ teaspoon of dried rosemary

For the steak

- 20 oz of flank steak, cut meat into 4 equal portions

- ½ cup of *chimichurri* (recipe included)

- ¼ cup of black pepper marinade (recipe included)

- 1 bunch of asparagus, remove the white parts

For the *sofrito*

- 1 Serrano chili

- $^1/_3$ cup of fresh and roughly chopped ginger

- $^1/_3$ cup of roughly chopped shallots

- ½ cup of extra-virgin olive oil

For the *chimichurri*

- ¾ cup of packed baby arugula

- ¼ cup of zero belly *sofrito* (recipe included)

- ½ bunch of fresh parsley

- 3 tablespoons of red wine vinegar

- ¼ teaspoon of kosher salt

- 2 cloves of garlic, minced

- ¼ teaspoon of ground black pepper

For the black pepper marinade

- 2 tablespoons of whole coriander seeds

- ½ tablespoon of whole cumin seeds

- 2 tablespoons of whole black peppercorns

- 6 cloves of garlic, skin removed

- 3 shallots, remove the skin then slice thinly

- 1 inch of fresh ginger, thinly sliced

- ¼ cup of extra-virgin olive oil

- ¼ cup of brown sugar

Cooking Directions:

1. Turn on the oven and set to 400°F or (200°C.)

2. Peel the skin from the potatoes and halve lengthwise. Cut each potato half into 6 wedges and place it in a large mixing bowl. Add in the olive oil, thyme and rosemary into the mixing bowl and mix until the potato wedges are coated evenly.

3. Prepare a nonstick sheet pan and place the potato wedges on top in a single layer. Place the sheet pan on the middle rack in the oven and bake for 30 minutes. Once done, the potatoes should be cooked through and the edges crisp.

4. Grind the cumin seeds, peppercorns and coriander seeds until the spices become very fine. Place the ground spices in a small food processor and add in the garlic, ginger, shallots, olive oil and brown sugar. Puree until the mixture becomes smooth.

5. Rub the black pepper marinade on both sides of the meat and marinate for a minimum of 10 minutes.

6. Prepare a grill pan and set over medium-high heat. Using tongs, place the steaks on the grill pan and let it sit for 4 minutes or until the meat has achieved nice grill marks. Turn the steak about the quarter on the same side and cook for another 4 minutes. Repeat the procedure when cooking the other side of the steaks.

7. After cooking the steaks, place them on serving plates and let rest. Then, add the asparagus on the grill pan. Cook and flip the asparagus until the vegetables become tender. Divide the potato wedges and asparagus into 4 servings and place it on the serving plates.

8. Remove the stem from the Serrano chili and cut in half. Remove the seeds from the chili and slice thinly. Place in a food processor and add in the shallots and ginger. Process until finely minced.

9. Prepare a saucepan and set over medium heat. Add the olive oil and the contents of the food processor. Lower the heat and cook for 8 minutes or until the shallots are soft. Remove from the heat and set aside.

10. Clean the food processor and add in the parsley and arugula. Pulse until the greens are well-chopped. Add the sofrito, red wine vinegar, garlic, kosher salt and black pepper into the food processor, and pulse until the ingredients are well-incorporated but still chunky.

11. Place 2 tablespoons of the chimichurri on top of each steak before serving.

This recipe is good for 4 servings.

Unbelievable Chili

Enjoy this chili recipe and warm your stomach on a chilly evening.

Ingredients:

- 1 tablespoon of olive oil

- 1 medium zucchini, diced

- 1 medium onion, minced

- ½ lb of *cremini* mushrooms, diced

- 1 red bell pepper, diced

- 1 medium carrot, diced

- 2 cloves of garlic, minced

- 2 canned chipotle peppers, chopped finely

- 1 can of whole peeled tomatoes

- 1 teaspoon of chili powder

- ½ teaspoon of dried oregano

- ¼ teaspoon of ground cumin

- 1 can of pinto beans, drained

- ½ avocado, sliced

- Salt

- Black pepper

Cooking Directions:

1. Prepare a pot and set over medium heat. Heat the olive oil.
2. Add the zucchini, onion, carrot, mushrooms, garlic and red bell pepper. Cook and stir frequently for 10 minutes or until the vegetables are lightly browned and soft.

3. Crush the tomatoes lightly using your fingers before adding into the pot. Then, add in the chili powder, chipotle peppers, oregano, cumin and pinto beans. Use salt and pepper to season accordingly. Stir and reduce the heat to low and let the soup simmer for 20 minutes.

4. Transfer into bowls and add an avocado slice on top before serving.

This recipe is good for 4 servings.

Burger Night and Day

Enjoy the ultimate burger party with this amazingly healthy recipe.

Ingredients:

- 1 lb of ground lean beef

- 1 teaspoon of freshly cracked pepper

- 1 teaspoon of salt

- 8 oz of mushrooms, sliced

- 4 hamburger buns (gluten-free)

- ½ teaspoon of extra-virgin olive oil

- 2 cups of arugula

- Ketchup

- Mustard

- ½ cup of caramelized onions

Cooking Directions:

1. Preheat grill.

2. Add the ground beef, salt and freshly cracked pepper in a mixing bowl. Combine the ingredients together and

form 4 burger patties. Be careful not to overwork the meat or pack the patties tightly as it may result to tough burgers.

3. Grill the burgers for 3 minutes and flip. Cook for another 3 minutes and set it aside. Toast the buns in the grill while still hot.

4. Prepare a pan and sauté the mushrooms in olive oil. Once the mushrooms become soft and the excess liquid is released, remove the mushrooms from the pan.

5. Divide the arugula equally into 4 portions and place it on top of the hamburger buns. Then, place the burger, mushroom and caramelized onion on top. Serve while still warm.

This recipe is good for 4 servings.

Dinosaur Salad

Craving for something light? This salad is heavy on the taste but light on your belly, perfect for lunch or dinner.

Ingredients:

- 2 cups of dinosaur kale, remove the ribs and chop

- 4 Kalamata olives, pitted and halved

- ¼ cup of cherry tomatoes, halved

- ¼ cup of artichoke hearts

- ⅛ red onion, diced

- ¼ cup of cooked chickpeas

- 2 tablespoons of walnuts

- Salt

- Black pepper

- 1 tablespoon of cider vinaigrette

Cooking Directions:

1. Massage and squeeze the kale for a few minutes before preparing the salad to make the vegetable tender.

2. Place the tomatoes, kale, artichoke hearts, olives, onion, chickpeas and walnuts in a salad bowl. Add in the cider vinaigrette, black pepper and salt, and toss to combine.

This recipe is good for 1 serving.

Grill, Grill, Grill

Grilling is a healthier way to cook meat and by using this recipe, you'll be sure to create a juicy and tasty meal.

Ingredients:

- 1 lb of flank steak

- 1 tablespoon of brown sugar

- ¼ cup of soy sauce (low sodium)

- ½ tablespoon of sesame oil

- 1 English cucumber, sliced thinly

- 3 tablespoons of rice wine vinegar

- Salt

- 2 cups of cooked brown rice

- 1 head of Bibb lettuce, separate the leaves

- Sriracha sauce and hoisin sauce

Cooking Directions:

1. Combine the brown sugar, sesame oil, soy sauce, 1 tablespoon of rice wine vinegar and flank steak in a mixing bowl. Cover the bowl with plastic wrap and marinate the meat in the refrigerator about 4 hours before cooking.

2. About 1 hour before cooking, combine the remaining vinegar, salt and cucumber in a small bowl. Set aside.

3. Prepare a cast-iron skillet and set over medium-high heat. Cook the steak for 4 minutes on each side. Once done, slice the steak thinly. Serve with the lettuce leaves, sriracha, hoisin and brown rice.

This recipe is good for 4 servings.

Salmon in Mystery Sauce

Take a break from meat and enjoy this mysterious salmon dish that will leave you wanting for more.

Ingredients:

- 2 teaspoons of extra-virgin olive oil

- ½ teaspoon of sugar

- ½ teaspoon of ground cumin

- ½ teaspoon of black pepper

- 4 salmon fillets

- ½ teaspoon of salt and a pinch

- ½ cup of non-fat Greek yogurt

- 1 scallion, trimmed then chopped finely

- 1 large pickling cucumber, seeded and peeled then diced

- 3 tablespoons of minced fresh parsley

- 8 oz of whole wheat orzo, prepare according to package directions

- 1 teaspoon of fresh lemon juice

Cooking Directions:

1. In a mixing bowl, combine the cumin, olive oil, black pepper, ½ teaspoon of salt and sugar. Stir until well-combined.

2. Prepare a baking sheet and line it with tin foil. Place the salmon in the baking sheet and brush the top with the oil mixture. Place the baking sheet in the refrigerator for 20 minutes.

3. Preheat broiler.
4. In a small bowl, combine the cucumber, yogurt, parsley, scallion, a pinch of salt and lemon juice. Mix until well-combined.

5. Broil the salmon for 10 minutes or until the center of the thickest part is barely opaque. Serve on top of the orzo with the yogurt sauce.

This recipe is good for 4 servings.

Zero Belly Penne

Satisfy your pasta cravings with this delicious zero belly pasta recipe.

Ingredients:

- Salt

- 12 oz of whole wheat penne

- 1 bunch of broccoli *rabe* or *rapini*

- 1 tablespoon of extra-virgin olive oil

- ½ medium red onion, sliced thinly

- 2 lean Italian turkey sausages, remove casings

- 1 clove of garlic, sliced

- 2 tablespoons of tomato paste

- Crushed red pepper flakes

- ¼ cup of ricotta (part-skim)

- 2 tablespoons of grated parmesan cheese

Cooking Directions:

1. Fill a large pot with water and add salt. Bring water to boil then, add the broccoli *rabe* and cook for about 4 minutes. Do not throw water once done.

2. Transfer the broccoli *rabe* in a colander and let it cool. Once cool enough to handle, slice the vegetable into bite-sized pieces.

3. Add the penne into the same pot where you cooked the broccoli and cook the pasta until al dente. Reserve ½ cup of the cooking water before draining the pasta.

4. Prepare a large skillet and set over medium heat. Add the onion, turkey sausages, a pinch of red pepper flakes, and garlic. Using a wooden spoon, crumble the sausages and cook for 5 minutes.

5. Add the chopped broccoli and cook for another 2 minutes.

6. Add the tomato paste and stir until the ingredients are properly combined. Cook for another minute.

7. Reduce the heat and add the pasta to the skillet. Toss until the ingredients are well-combined. Add the reserved cooking water if the pasta seems dry. Add in the parmesan cheese and ricotta and remove the pan from the heat. Toss until well-combined. Serve while still warm.

This recipe is good for 4 servings.

Chapter 5: Desserts

Chocolate Bark

Having a stressful day at work? No worries. Now, you can eat chocolate even without excuses! This high-fiber chocolate dessert will surely satisfy your chocolate cravings any time of the day.

Ingredients:

- 10 oz of semisweet chocolate chips

- ¼ cup of raw *pepitas*, dry roasted and cooled

- ½ cup of dried tart cherries

- ¼ cup of raw almonds, dry roasted and coarsely chopped

Cooking Directions:

1. Turn on the oven and set to 350°F or 175°C.

2. Prepare a baking pan and line it with parchment paper. Place the chocolate chips on top of the parchment paper and spread until it forms a rectangle about 8 inches long.

3. Place the baking pan in the oven and bake for 3 minutes. The chocolate should start to melt at this point.

4. Transfer the baking pan on a cooling rack and use an offset spatula to spread the melting chocolate into a smooth rectangle. Sprinkle the cherries, *pepitas* and almonds on top.

5. Refrigerate for a minimum of 30 minutes. Transfer the parchment paper on a plate and break the chocolate bark into small rectangles.

This recipe is good for 10 servings.

Chocolate Cake

Now you can indulge on a piece of heaven, one slice at a time.

Ingredients:

- 6 oz of semisweet chocolate chips

- ½ cup of granulated sugar

- ¼ cup of maple syrup

- 3 large eggs

- ¼ teaspoon of kosher salt

- ½ cup of unsweetened cocoa powder

- 1 teaspoon of vanilla extract

- Olive oil cooking spray

- Fresh berries

Cooking Directions:

1. Turn on oven and set to 350°F or 175°C. Prepare an 8-inch spring form pan and lightly coat with olive oil cooking spray.

2. Line the bottom with parchment paper and spray again with olive oil.

3. In a small saucepan, melt the chocolate together with the maple syrup over low heat. Once the chocolate

melts, add the sugar and stir for 2 minutes or until the sugar dissolves completely.

4. Remove the saucepan from the heat and whisk in one egg at a time.

5. Using a sieve, sift the cocoa powder into the saucepan. Whisk into the chocolate mixture and make sure to avoid any lumps. Add salt and vanilla extract and mix again.

6. Pour the cake batter into the spring form pan and bake for about 25 minutes or until the cake is firm.

7. Cut into 8 equal slices and garnish with the fresh berries. Serve while still warm.

This recipe is good for 8 servings.

Black Forest Twist

We've put on a twist on a signature dessert to create a satisfying and guilt-free treat.

Ingredients:

- 2 ¼ cups of finely ground almond meal

- ½ teaspoon of baking soda

- ¼ cup of unsweetened cocoa powder

- ½ cup of coconut oil, melted

- 2 large eggs

- ½ cup of light brown sugar

- ¾ cup of semisweet chocolate chips

- Olive oil cooking spray

- ½ cup of dried tart cherries, chopped roughly

-

Cooking Directions:

1. Turn on the oven and set to 350°F or 175°C.

2. Prepare 2 sheet pans and line each with parchment paper, then spray with olive oil cooking spray.

3. In a mixing bowl, mix the cocoa powder, baking soda and almond meal.

4. In another bowl, whisk together the coconut oil, eggs and light brown sugar. Gradually add in the almond meal mixture into the bowl and stir until properly incorporated. Add in the chocolate chips and cherries and stir.

5. Take a tablespoon of cookie dough and arrange it on top of a sheet pan. Leave at least 2 inches of space in between cookie dough.

6. Place the sheet pans in the oven and bake for 12 minutes. Remove the sheet pan from the oven and wait for 2 minutes before transferring the cookies on a cooling rack.

This recipe makes 24 cookies.

Peanut Butter and Choco Truffles

Munch on this easy-to-make and guilt-free dessert at home or on the go.

Ingredients:

- 6 oz of semisweet chocolate chips

- ½ cup of natural creamy peanut butter (no salt added)

- ¼ cup of unsweetened almond milk

Cooking Directions:

1. In a microwave-safe bowl, add in the almond milk and chocolate chips. Microwave until the chocolate melts. Make sure to stir every 30 seconds.

2. Once the chocolate melts, whisk in the peanut butter until the mixture becomes smooth. Cover the bowl with plastic wrap and refrigerate until the mixture is firm.

3. Using a spoon, scoop marble-sized truffles from the mixture and roll into a ball. The mixture should be enough for 20 truffles.

4. Transfer the truffles on a tray lined with wax paper and chill until firm. Serve while still cold.

This recipe makes 20 truffles.

2-Ingredient Blackberry Ice Cream

The hardest part about this recipe is waiting for the bananas to freeze. Other than that, you are good to go.

Ingredients:

- 6 pieces overripe bananas, placed in freezer-safe bags, frozen in their skins for 24 hours

- 2 cups frozen blackberries, thawed lightly

-

Preparations:

1. Peel bananas and roughly chop.

2. Place these along with blackberries in blender. Pulse and process until relatively smooth. Scrape down sides often.

3. Scoop equal portions into tiny sundae glasses. Serve immediately.

This recipe makes 4 servings.

Green Smoothie Popsicles

Consuming popsicles on hot days is always great, but you can also add this recipe to your after-dinner treats.

Ingredients:

- ¼ packed cup raisins

- 1 large grapefruit, pulp only, deseeded

- 1 large overripe banana, peeled, chopped

- 1 tablespoon raw chia seeds

- 1 large kiwi fruit, peeled, quartered

- 1 small red delicious apple, peeled, cored, cubed

- 1 heaping cup fresh pineapple chunks, cored, cubed

- 2 handfuls fresh baby spinach, rinsed, spun-dried

Preparations:

1. Place ingredients in blender. Pulse and process until relatively smooth. Scrape down sides often.

2. Pour smoothie into popsicle moulds. Freeze solid. Unmould. Serve.

This recipe makes 10 to 12 popsicles.

Red Smoothie Popsicles

These popsicles have a bit of tartness with a hint of sweetness, but packed to the gills with vitamins and minerals. These also provide a bit of chew with fresh pomegranate seeds.

Ingredients:

- 1 cup frozen raspberries, thawed lightly

- 1 large grapefruit, pulp only, deseeded

- 1 large blood orange, pulp only, deseeded

- 1 large overripe banana, peeled, chopped

- 1 cup frozen cranberries, thawed lightly

- 1 large pomegranate, seeds whacked out, include juices

Preparations:

1. Place small pinches of pomegranate seeds into popsicle moulds. Set aside.

2. Pour remaining ingredients in blender. Pulse and process until relatively smooth. Scrape down sides often.

3. Pour smoothie into popsicle moulds with pomegranate seeds. Freeze solid. Un-mould. Serve.

This recipe makes 10 to 12 popsicles.

Green Giant

Adding some greens into your diet will boost your health while helping you lose weight.

Ingredients:

- ¼ cup of apple juice (no sugar added)

- ½ scoop of vanilla protein powder (plant-based)

- ¼ cup of water

- ½ Bosc pear, chopped

- ½ frozen banana

- ½ cup of loosely packed baby spinach

- ¼ ripe avocado

Preparations:

1. Add in the pear, banana, avocado and baby spinach in a blender. Blend until the ingredients are well-incorporated.

2. Add in the apple juice, protein powder and water. Blend until the mixture becomes smooth.

3. Transfer smoothie in a serving glass and consume immediately.

This recipe makes 1 generous serving.

Vanilla *Chai*

Whether you're having a busy or lazy afternoon, this drink will not only relax your senses but satisfy your cravings as well.

Ingredients:

- ¼ cup of unsweetened almond milk

- ½ scoop of vanilla protein powder (plant-based)

- ¼ cup of *chai* tea, brewed then chilled

- ½ frozen banana

- ½ tablespoon of unsalted natural almond butter

- ½ teaspoon of ground cinnamon

- Water

Preparations:

1. Add in the almond milk, protein powder, *chai* tea, banana, almond butter and cinnamon in a blender.

2. Process until smooth and well-combined. Add water if needed.

3. Serve and consume immediately.

This recipe makes 1 generous serving.

Peanut Butter Cup

A zero belly dessert that is better and healthier alternative to your usual store-bought peanut butter cup sweets.

Ingredients:

- ½ cup of unsweetened almond milk

- 1 tablespoon of unsweetened cocoa powder

- 1 tablespoon of chocolate protein powder (plant-based)

- ½ frozen banana

- Water

- ½ tablespoon of natural unsalted peanut butter

Preparations:

1. Combine the almond milk, cocoa powder, protein powder, banana and peanut butter in a food processor.

2. Blend until well-combined. Add water to achieve preferred consistency.

3. Serve and consume immediately.

This recipe makes 1 generous serving.

Blueberry Blast

Complete your blueberry breakfast ensemble with this blueberry smoothie delight.

Ingredients:

- ½ cup of unsweetened almond milk

- ½ cup of frozen blueberries

- 1 scoop of vanilla protein powder (plant-based)

- ½ tablespoon of natural unsalted almond butter

- Water

Preparations:

1. Add the almond milk, blueberries, protein powder and almond butter in a blender. Mix until smooth.

2. Add water to achieve desired consistency. Serve and consume as soon as possible.

This recipe makes 1 generous serving.

Strawbanana Smoothie

Get a dose of yummy goodness all day, every day with this amazing smoothie recipe.

Ingredients:

- 1 scoop of protein powder (plant-based)

- ¼ frozen banana

- $1/3$ cup of frozen strawberries

- ½ teaspoon of almond butter

- Water

- ½ cup of unsweetened almond milk

Preparation:

1. Add the protein powder, banana, strawberries, almond butter and almond milk in a blender. Process until the mixture becomes smooth to drink. Add more water if necessary.

2. Serve and consume immediately.

This recipe makes 1 generous serving.

Apple Pie Smoothie

Lots of people love apple pies. But did you know that many of its individual components like are fat-burners as well? Load up on this drink either as a meal replacement for lunch, or (in reduced portions) as a refreshing snack.

Ingredients:

- ½ cup raw cashew nuts, soaked in water overnight, drained well

- 1 cup unsweetened cashew milk

- 1 cup ice cubes or shaved ice

- 1 large overripe frozen banana, peeled, cubed

- 1 tsp. cinnamon powder

- 2 large red Fuji apples, peeled, cored, chopped

- dash of ginger powder

- dash of nutmeg powder

- ½ cup raisins

- pinch of green *stevia,* optional

Preparation:

1. Pour ingredients into blender. Process until smooth.

2. Serve and consume immediately.

This recipe makes 2 generous servings.

Virgin Piña Colada

Alcohol is off the menu, of course. But that doesn't mean that you can't enjoy a glass of tweaked out piña colada on a hot day.

Ingredients:

- 2 cans, 6 ounces each crushed pineapples, do not drain

- 1 can 15 ounces coconut cream

- 1 cup ice cubes or shaved ice

- mint leaves for garnish

- 1 large overripe frozen banana, peeled, cubed

- pinch of green *stevia,* optional

Preparation:

1. Except for mint leaves, pour remaining ingredients into blender. Process until smooth.

2. Pour in tall glasses. Garnish with mint leaves. Serve.

This recipe makes 2 generous servings or 3 smaller ones.

Bonus Chapter: Tea-time!

Did you know that tea also plays a major role in breaking down body fats? To get you started in the healthy habit of drinking tea (if you're not already), here are some suggestions on where to start.

White Tea
Try these brands: The Republic of Tea, Twinings, Celestial Seasonings Sleepytime

White tea breaks down the body's stored fats and at the same time, prevents the formation of new fat cells. It also helps the liver turn stored fat into energy and release fat from cells.

Barberry
Try these brands: TeaHaven, TerraVita

According to Chinese researches, Barberry contains berberin, a fat-burning chemical that can prevent weight gain and insulin resistance for people who consume a high-fat diet.

Pu-erh Tea
Try these brands: Uncle Lee's Tea, Numi Organic Tea

This Chinese tea has been proven to deflate flat cells, resulting to a significant reduction in belly flab. Drink every morning and pair it with the recipes above for better results.

Oolong Tea
Try these brands: Stash, Bigelow

This traditional Chinese tea has been proven to aid a person's digestion and increase metabolism. Aside from that, this tea also helps keep cholesterol levels in check to keep the heart healthy.

Rooibos Tea

Try these brands: Teavana, Celestial Seasonings

This sweet red tea is a powerful fat-melter. It also prevents the formation of new fat cells. It also helps in digestion for faster metabolism and burns stubborn belly fat.

Conclusion

Thank you again for downloading this book, *"Zero Belly Cookbook - Achieve your body goals without sacrificing your enjoyment for food!"*

Losing weight doesn't mean that you have to spend most of your waking hours eating raw celery and carrot sticks – or what other people might consider as "rabbit food." There are ways on how you can enjoy your favorite meals, at relatively large volumes, *and* still lose weight at the same time. You just need to follow some basic guidelines (as stated in the first chapter of this book.)

Hopefully, by trying out some of the recipes in this book, you will discover how to tweak your favorite recipes so that these work well with your weight loss endeavor. Who knows? You might even discover new favorites as you go along?

Finally, if you enjoyed this book, then I'd like to ask you for a favor, would you be kind enough to leave a good review for this book on Amazon? It'd be greatly appreciated!

Click here to leave a review for this book on Amazon!

Thank you and good luck!

32988744R10059

Made in the USA
Middletown, DE
25 June 2016